Reverse Liver Cirrhosis in 90 Days
By
Nirmal Raghavan

Published by: Kindle Direct Publishing July 2018
Ancient Cure Series Book 2

Disclaimer: This treatment or diet plan is not a substitute for medical attention, treatment, examination, advice or diagnosis and is not intended to provide a clinical diagnosis nor take the place of proper medical advice from a fully qualified medical practitioner. You should, before you act or use any of this information, consider the appropriateness of this information having regard to your situation and needs. You are responsible for consulting a suitable medical professional before using any of the information contained in this ebook, before trying any treatment or taking any course of action that may directly or indirectly affect your health or well-being.

Contents

About

Nirmal Raghavan is a pharmaceutical researcher from India. He has over ten years of experience in pharmaceutical and cosmetic industries with research, synthesis, phytochemical extraction, and quality. By early 2010 his interest shifted to natural cures, and over the years, he explored the wisdom of ancient Indian seers through various available resources. In this 'Ancient cure series,' he substantiates his findings with contemporary scientific research of gut microbiome and its direct relation to various diseases. The book offers you a completely different perspective in dealing with and treating liver diseases.

Introduction

Liver cirrhosis is one of the major causes of death worldwide over the past few decades. What is the leading cause of this disease? Is this curable by any medication? Well, these are the questions many a ask when they come across such a situation. The age-old story of alcoholism, heredity or unknown factors are the leading causes says the scientific community. This is true when you see things from a pharmaceutical research perspective. But if you dig deeper into a microbial level, things are a bit different and, indeed, there is a cure for liver cirrhosis. When I say, there is a cure it is an intensive procedure that you need to undergo to get rid of this. Recent researches are pretty close to the real cause as now they say dysbiosis is the primary cause of liver cirrhosis. Does that mean the age-old story of alcoholism, heredity or unknown factors has nothing to do with it? Yes, they do, but dysbiosis is something precise, and by knowing this in detail, the condition is treatable. The primary stage of liver cirrhosis is fatty liver. Over time this progresses to liver fibrosis, and that leads to liver cirrhosis. If life doesn't end there, this can lead to liver cancer eventually. These are external manifestations of an internal problem which now we call dysbiosis.

The entire cure procedure and its scientific background have a deep-rooted base on ancient wisdom from the Indian subcontinent, followed by the seers with dysbiosis as its backend, they treated this condition with food restrictions, herbal medicines, and diet. They make herbal medicine as a medium to rejuvenate the beneficial microbes mainly across the gut and the whole system, thereby expelling pathogens gradually over a period. According to them, the procedure will get its full effect if you organize your life with prompt daily routines and practicing meditation techniques to calm your mind. They reckon this is indispensably important as both mind and body should work together to cure the disease. If everything goes fine, you can achieve this in as early as 90 days. I tried my best to present the subject with a Q&A session below which will help you deeply understand the subject.

1. Dysbiosis and Liver Diseases

What is dysbiosis?

Dysbiosis is an impaired microbiota across any part of the body, for example, skin dysbiosis or gut dysbiosis is an imbalance in the microbial equilibrium occurs at that part of the body. But when you say dysbiosis in general, this means an imbalance in the gut microbiome – few kilograms of microbes living on the mucous membrane of the small intestine and down below.

What is a healthy gut microbiome and what is its relation to the liver?

A healthy gut microbiome is a diverse colony of different microbes that live in the gut that processes the food we eat to micronutrients. When pathogens get into this system and colonize, things would take a different turn. They process food not to nutrients but toxins. These toxins will affect the regeneration process happening across the system. When the cells don't get enough nutrients to regenerate, a situation occurs that we call degeneration.

In the case of the liver, this degeneration may lead to liver cirrhosis as overtime scar cells replace normal cells. But, before cirrhosis, if there is a healthy gut microbiome, the liver will regenerate entirely in as early as six weeks.

What are pathogens and what is their role in the gut microbiome?

In the simple picture, pathogens are microbes that produce toxins instead of micronutrients with the food we eat. I wouldn't call them pathogens, but they act like pathogens only when they are in our system which means they got a different role in nature. Unlike infectious bacteria or virus, these pathogens can thrive in the system without being noticed by the immune system. They get into our system and flourish since we feed them on a daily basis with food containing less fortifying nutrients. When the body receives fewer nutrients, it won't regenerate at the same pace as it would, this happens with the liver in liver cirrhosis.

What leads to fatty liver and ultimately to liver cirrhosis from a microbial perspective?

Unwanted fat settlements in the liver cells are the primary stage of liver disease. This by itself is a result of a microbial imbalance in the

gut(chapter 4). While this happens, there would
be a change in the microbiota across the liver
system like the microbial changes with plaque
formation in the arteries. Eventually, this change
proceeds to inflammation of the liver and may
even get further foreign settlements. End of the
day, fewer nutrients for liver regeneration and
the equilibrium of liver regeneration shifts
towards the left side. At this stage, we can see
the difference in the liver function test, and we
call it a liver disease.

Death of liver cells   ↔ Regeneration of liver cells

If you provide with enough natural nutrients,
you can maintain the equilibrium again, and if
you colonize beneficial microbes that produce
these micronutrients, the liver can come back to
normal.
But in the case of liver cirrhosis, scar tissues
takes the place of normal liver cells. Hence every
regeneration is again a scar cell. In this extreme
case, we need to reintroduce beneficial microbes
that can supply enough nutrients with the help
of a fortified herbal media, normal liver cells will
replace these scar cells, and that is the basis of
this treatment.

Could you elaborate gut microbiome in detail?

The mucous lining of our gut is being colonized
by 700 to 1000 species of microbes which
include bacteria, yeast, archaea, fungi and many
more. These all thrive on the specific food we eat
and at particular temperatures. 60 % of feces are
microorganisms, and only the rest is solid matter
and water. When we eat food, these microbes
convert it into micronutrients. But when
pathogens get into the system, they produce
toxins instead. We wouldn't recognize this until
the number of pathogens reasonably increased.
When this happens, any of the specific nutrients
needed for a particular organ's regeneration
doesn't get processed at the same pace. Again, if
the number of pathogens increases, the waste
they produce accumulates in the body and this
can make our system prone to more and more
different pathogens. The whole process
wouldn't happen in a day or a few months. This
process takes years or even decades to occur. If
favorable situations arise, this can happen in as
short a few months.

**If it were pathogens why liver and why not
other organs?**
Indeed this is one of the critical questions I
initially had and is a bit hard to understand.

A reasonable explanation is given by one of the seers of south India as he reckons this could happen by two chances. The primary being due to the consumption of alcohol or other drugs, the person loses much of the beneficial gut flora that provides specific nutrients for liver regeneration(chapter 4). The second reason is local colonization of pathogens across liver vessels that converts the vital nutrients for liver regeneration to toxins. Recent research shows a similar explanation[i].

2. Food as a Medium

Which all foods cause these pathogens to multiply?

Any processed food would be a suitable medium for pathogens. When we process food, it loses its natural nutrients like vitamins, alkaloids, flavonoids, carotenoids, polyphenols, etc. that we generally call as phytochemicals. When these natural agents do not protect food, pathogens can quickly grow in them – i.e., this food will convert to an excellent medium for any of the many pathogens.

Why are processed foods not recommended for liver diseases?

When we process food either by heating or other chemical methods, the food will lose many vital phytochemicals. Of the processed foods, fried foods are the worst. When we fry, food temperature can rise to over 200°celcius, and many vital nutrients like vitamins disintegrate below this temperature. Finally, what you get is food with unprotected carbohydrates and proteins that act as a suitable medium for pathogens. It is not the oils that are bad but the protective nutrients disintegrate while boiling or processing them makes them bad. On the other hand boiled food retain some of the nutrients present in the food but nothing much in comparison with raw food. Same with the case of food processed with chemicals or increasing their shelf-life with preservatives. Not many beneficial microbes multiply in chemically modified or processed foods. Preservatives are meant to stop microbial growth. Hence, any use of them in food wouldn't help us in any way.

Are processed foods bad for everybody?

If you have a healthy gut flora, you don't need to worry about any food. Just like most of the children can eat any junk food without any problems. When you grow older, the situation would be different, as pathogens get into your system and start multiplying and colonizing extensively across the gut or other local sites and would give you specific symptoms. Pathogenic colonization might take many years in many cases but would be as short as months in a favorable situation. The situation goes favorable depending on a few parameters for pathogenic growth.

What are the parameters controlling microbial growth?
Any microbial growth needs three things to thrive and colonize. They are primarily the

microbes, then the medium to grow and the
 right temperature for growth. Here, this is the
favorable situation mentioned in the above
question. For pathogens, if they get unprotected
food – food without many natural nutrients,
they would multiply with ease. On the other
hand, if there are natural phytochemicals, the
food gets protected, and beneficial ones increase.
But, if you expose to cold weather, cold rooms or
cold foods, even if you're eating good food,
things favor pathogens as many pathogens
prefer lower temperatures to flourish and they
get stronger to process even protected food to
some extent.

Typically what happens with every microbial
species is, when they break down the food, they
generate a temperature for their optimum
growth. The way they disintegrate food is to
create a waste that can be favorable for their
growth. Hence each species of microbes have
different temperatures for their optimal growth.
When microbes produce waste that are toxins to
our system, we call them pathogens and when it
is micronutrients then beneficial microbes. If the
amount of pathogens in your system is on the
increase you are prone to further diseases as the
waste of pathogens would favor many other
specific pathogens to grow in your system.

3. Preparation and Treatment

Is this a diet plan or herbal medication?

We need both in this condition. Before I take you to all those steps, I would like you to understand that this is an intensive treatment plan. You need to take immense care as you know liver cirrhosis is a bit complicated. You may be having esophageal varices, bacterial peritonitis or hepatic encephalopathy. In those extreme cases, you need to be entirely under the supervision of your gastroenterologist. As you know, with the herbal medications and diet what we would be aiming for is, bring up the number of beneficial microbes. The procedure would take many days to see any better results. If everything goes fine, you can see changes in as early as 15 days to a month.

How does this treatment work?
The treatment is no miracle cure but based on pure scientific background. Its all about herbal medications as a medium to increase the number of beneficial microbes and not feeding the pathogens. The procedure continues for three months following the same diet and medications to make beneficial microbes colonize your system that they can provide your system with

enough nutrients for proper regeneration of the
liver cells. You can see a better shift after 45 to
60 days of treatment when the pace of beneficial
ones colonizing the gut increases and you can
feel the change. Proper colonization of microbes
can take anywhere between 90 to 180 days. 90
days is the minimum when everything goes
smooth and nice.

Are there any preparations for this treatment?

If alcohol is the cause of liver cirrhosis, it is
mandatory that you need to stop it completely,
so you do with smoking. Completely avoid
meat, fish, refined sugar and egg for the whole
treatment period. All these are good mediums
for pathogens to thrive. Since this is an intensive
procedure, you should only take what the
procedure recommends. If you follow other
foods, you may feed pathogens in between, and
their colonies will go stronger.

End-stage liver disease patients would be very
tired and bedridden most of the time. They may
have a distended abdomen, portal hypertension,
bacterial peritonitis, hepatic encephalopathy,
esophageal varices, etc. These are all various
manifestations of the underlying cirrhosis.
During ancient times, the treatment would have
started at earlier stages that it wouldn't progress

further or they take only potent medicated foods that the symptoms subside fast at any stages of the disease. Here with the symptoms mentioned above, treatment should be continued with your medical practitioner to bring all those symptoms under control. You can take these medications and diet plan while on treatment but again never mix your normal medications with herbal ones. Always keep an hour or more than an hour, between the two.

The base of the whole procedure is an herbal media as used by ancient Indian seers and they use these entirely to extend their lives exclusively for spiritual pursuits. Hence the primary thing they follow is organizing their lives. Once you start feeling a bit better and able to do your daily chores by yourself, organize your life, i.e., waking up, cleaning yourself, eating food, sleeping, etc. should be prompt. An unclean mind or body produces toxins that facilitate pathogens to thrive. The same is as important as the herbal medicines and the diet plan you follow in this procedure.

What is the procedure?

There are two procedures for you to choose from.
The procedures composed of two steps
 (1) Herbal medicines
 (2) Diet plan

Procedure 1

Step 1

Herbal medicine consists of capsules of the following herbs which are available online.

1. Kutki(Picrorhiza kurroa)
2. Bhringraj(Eclipta prostrata)
3. Chanca Piedra(Phyllanthus niruri)
4. Punarnava(Boerhavia diffusa)
5. Daruharidra (Berberis aristata)
6. Guduchi (Tinospora cordifolia)

When you buy these herbs, please make sure that these are the dried **herbs alone** and not any ingredients added to it especially no preservatives or any other chemicals. 400mg to 500 mg capsules of each above herbs should be taken two times a day 10 to 15 minutes after food morning and evening. After a couple of weeks, once you are immune to it, you can take this three times a day after food with suitable intervals.

One Indian gooseberry (frozen ones available at many Indian stores)grounded with an inch or half an inch piece of fresh turmeric should be taken on an empty stomach early morning, noon and night before your dinner. On early morning just after taking this do not eat or drink anything for 45mins to 1.5hrs to digest it properly. After 15 to 20 days replace fresh turmeric with less than 1/4th teaspoon of turmeric powder. Fresh turmeric is too strong and may limit the proliferation of beneficial microbes but helps in reducing pathogens for a short term.

Step 2

Ingredients

Brown Basmati rice
Moringa oleifera powder
Organic extra virgin coconut oil or organic extra virgin olive oil
Turmeric powder

Cook basmati rice with half a teaspoon of turmeric(for 2 cups of basmati). Mix this with extra virgin coconut oil(just enough oil to mix properly) and half a teaspoon of moringa powder. Make different portions and consume it every two hours. Most of the cirrhosis patients wouldn't have any appetite at all. Also, it's hard for them to digest a lot of foods at a time. Hence always take small portions but many times a day or as your appetite.

You can add freshly cut raw veggies with the above rice. Veggies can be carrots, cabbage, beets, lettuce, cucumber, onions and many more.

Pineapple can be taken for the first week but not after that. Pineapple contains an enzyme called bromelain that washes off the mucous layer in your gut where all these microbes colonized. Hence it is good for the first week to clean a bit but not after that. We build up beneficial ones after this so avoid it completely after the first week.

If available completely grass-fed raw milk would be an excellent food that you need to take at this stage. When Spanish scientists analyzed breast milk in 2012 [ii], they found 700 to 1000 species of microbes in it. Breastfeeding is the time when the mother transfers her immunity to the child. Moreover, the food we eat turns out to be the milk, and that's why the composition and nutrition of milk changes[iii]. Hence, completely grass-fed milk contains only beneficial bacteria since no pathogens can thrive in rich phytochemical grass juice that comes out as milk. You can also do your research on grass-fed cows as they have very very rare diseases and have a very long lifespan. Raw milk should be taken within an hour of milking for best results. Refrigerated raw milk changes the composition over days till it completely spoils on a particular day. Although it seems like a spontaneous process, low-temperature microbes multiplying in it slowly and finally spoiling it. Not many beneficial ones grow in low temperatures as detailed in chapter two.

In saying that, since you don't have enough bacteria in your gut to process raw milk, this will take a few weeks for you to increase their counts. For a start, take 2 to three ounces two to three times a day and then increase the amount slowly when you feel confident to handle more. Otherwise, it would be hard for you to digest it. You may get an upset stomach.

If you can't get grass-fed raw milk, a glass of pasteurized milk of jersey cow boiled with $1/4^{th}$ of a teaspoon of turmeric powder(boiling gets curcumin- the active ingredient of turmeric into milk solids) should be taken three to four times a day. Add a pinch of moringa powder when it cools down a bit. Instead of water, you can drink this. Since protein intake is less with this diet, this would be a good substitute to boost up your albumin levels. Sprouted lentils are also good if you want to add with your diet.

You can take green tea with a bit of organic unfiltered and unheated honey. Add the honey after the tea cools down a bit to retain as much as fortifying nutrients.

Avoid glycaemic fruits like bananas. Apples in moderation are good but avoid the sour ones. Avoid all sour fruits. Pomegranate is good if you can get it. Completely avoid canned foods during this treatment. Also, stay away from all kinds of energy drinks and soft drinks.

Procedure 2

Step 1

Step 1 is the same as the step1 in procedure 1.

Step2

Raw veggie sandwiches made out of whole grain bread or multigrain bread with organic grass-fed butter as a spread(don't use any other spread- you wouldn't get protection if the processing of the spread by any other means). You can use all sliced raw veggies including onion, tomato, carrot, cucumber, beets, lettuce, spinach with a pinch of salt(salt should be limited or avoided if possible) and black pepper. Sprinkle moringa powder and turmeric powder on your veggies for best results.

Fruits, drinks and all other eatables are as same as procedure 1.

Juicing

Fresh juices of amla, bitter gourd, celery etc would be beneficial if you can take it in small amounts and increasing the volume over weeks. To start with one or to ounces two to three times a day would be fine. This is very important since your gut might not have enough beneficial microbes to process fresh fruits and veggies.

You may get an upset stomach or bloating sensation if you consume more. But over weeks you can achieve this. The same should be followed for all raw veggies and fruits if you can't handle it with the digestion process. Only fresh juice with little bit of unprocessed(unfiltered and unheated) honey if you cant handle the strong taste.

4. Scientific Evidence and Facts

Where is the evidence of these claims?

There is plenty of evidence to substantiate these claims. I would like to provide you some established facts which are easily available over the internet. There are heaps of research works published in many reputed international journals but only a few are quoted here for your reference.

1. A study conducted by M. Minemura and Y. Shimizu titled **'Gut microbiota and liver diseases'** reveals the close relation of liver diseases with gut microbiota is published in 'World Journal of Gastroenterology' Feb 14, 2015, pages 1691-1702.

Abstract of the study
Several studies revealed that gut microbiota are associated with various human diseases, e.g., metabolic diseases, allergies, gastroenterological diseases, and liver diseases. The liver can be greatly affected by changes in gut microbiota due to the entry of gut bacteria or their metabolites into the liver through the portal vein, and the liver-gut axis is important to

understand the pathophysiology of several liver diseases, especially non-alcoholic fatty liver disease and hepatic encephalopathy. Moreover, gut microbiota play a significant role in the development of alcoholic liver disease and hepatocarcinogenesis. Based on these previous findings, trials using probiotics have been performed for the prevention or treatment of liver diseases. In this review, we summarize the current understanding of the changes in gut microbiota associated with various liver diseases, and we describe the therapeutic trials of probiotics for those diseases.

2. Another study conducted by C.Acharya, MBBS and J. Bajaj, MD, MS titled "**Gut Microbiota and Complications of Liver Disease**' shed light to dysbiosis and how this dysbiosis impact liver disease and how can an altered gut microbiota plays an important role in liver cirrhosis and its modulation to prevent disease progression changes. This has been published in 'Gastroenterology Clinics of North America', Volume 46, Issue 1, March 2017, Pages 155-169.

Abstract of the study

The epidemic of chronic liver disease and how to combat its complications has been a challenging aspect for many years. New laboratory techniques have made analysis of the human intestinal microbiome easier and also more detailed. With insight into dysbiosis and how this dysbiosis impacts liver disease, scientists have new targets in the intestine and liver. Dysbiosis is associated with endotoxemia and propagates liver injury in NASH and alcoholic cirrhosis. The composition of the microbiota changes with the development of cirrhosis and decompensation. Apart from microbes, the role that bile acids play in this arena are also being discovered and newer treatments like FXR receptor agonists are coming into the picture. Altered gut microbiota plays an important role in cirrhosis and its modulation to prevent disease progression changes, and concomitantly bile acid physiology must be regulated or augmented to help prevent cirrhosis and its complications.

3. Yet another study conducted by M S Zamparelli, A Rocco, D Compare and G Nardone published an article titled **"The gut microbiota: A new potential driving force in liver cirrhosis and hepatocellular carcinoma"** in 'United European Gastroenterology Journal' , Published on May 8, 2017, Volume 5,Issue:7, page(s): 944-953.

Abstract of the study

The gut microbiota has recently been recognized as a major environmental factor in the

pathophysiology of many human diseases.
The anatomical and function connection existing between gut and liver provides the theoretical basis to assume the liver is a major target for gut microbes. In the last decades, numerous studies reported an altered composition of gut microbiota in patients with liver cirrhosis and a progressively marked dysbiosis with worsening of the liver disease. The risk of developing hepatocellular carcinoma, the deadliest complication of liver cirrhosis, is widely variable among cirrhotic patients, thus suggesting a complexity of genetic and environmental factors implicated in hepatocarcinogenesis. Gut microbiota is now emerging as a plausible candidate to explain this variability. In this manuscript, we review the human and the experimental evidence supporting the potential implication of gut microbiota in the promotion, progression, and complication of liver disease.

4. Another study conducted by H Fukui published under the title '**Gut Microbiome-based Therapeutics in Liver Cirrhosis: Basic Consideration for the Next Step**' in 'Journal of Clinical and Translational Hepatology', Published online: June 29, 2017

Abstract of the study
Infections account for significant morbidity and mortality in liver cirrhosis and most are related

to the gut microbiome. Fecal dysbiosis, characterized by an overgrowth of potentially pathogenic bacteria and a decrease in autochthonous non-pathogenic bacteria, becomes prominent with the progression of liver cirrhosis. In cirrhotic patients, disruption of the intestinal barrier causes intestinal hyperpermeability (i.e. leaky gut), which is closely related to gut dysmotility, dysbiosis, and small intestinal bacterial overgrowth and may induce pathological bacterial translocation. Although the involved microbial taxa are somewhat different between the cirrhotic patients from the East and the West, the common manifestation of a shortage of bacteria that contribute to the production of short-chain fatty acids and secondary bile acids may facilitate intestinal inflammation, leaky gut, and gut dysbiosis. Translocated endotoxin and bacterial DNA are capable of provoking potent inflammation and affecting the metabolic and hemodynamic systems, which may ultimately enhance the progression of liver cirrhosis and its various complications, such as hepatic encephalopathy (HE), variceal bleeding, infection, and renal disturbances. Among studies on the microbiome-based therapeutics, findings of probiotic effects on HE have been contradictory in spite of several supportive results. However, the effects of synbiotics and prebiotics are substantially documented. The background of their effectiveness should be evaluated again in relation to the cirrhosis-related changes in gut microbiome and their metabolic effects. Strict indications for the antibiotic rifaximin remain unestablished, although its effect is promising, improving HE and other complications with little influence on microbial populations. The final goal of microbiome-based therapeutics is to adjust the gut-liver axis to the maximal benefit of cirrhotic patients, with the aid of evolving metagenomic and metabolomic analyses.

I strongly believe the above articles in reputed journals would give you enough information on the direct relationship between gut microbes and liver cirrhosis.
Now, I would like to shed some light on the pathology of liver cirrhosis on the intake of herbal medicines

1. A Study conducted by M Hong 1, S Li et al under the title '**Current Status of Herbal Medicines in Chronic Liver Disease Therapy: The Biological Effects, Molecular Targets and Future Prospects**' published in 'International Journal of Molecular Sciences, Volume 16, issue 12 sheds some light on the inefficiency of synthetic medicines in treating chronic liver diseases over herbal medicines.

The conclusion of this article is (available online)
The current review provides a detailed and
updated description of the most widely used
herbal medicine and herbal formulas used in
alleviating chronic liver disease. _It has been clearly
described that medicinal plants and phytochemicals
can treat chronic liver disease by inhibiting oxidative
damage, suppressing fibrogenesis, eliminating virus
infection, and preventing or inhibiting tumor growth._
_For some medicinal plants, the active components
still need to be further confirmed._

**Though some of the herbs in my book are
mentioned in the above article, I would like to
provide more evidence on the herbs prescribed
in my book.**

Moringa Oleifera

An article published by AA Hamza in 'Food and
chemical toxicology', Volume 48, Issue 1,
January 2010, Pages 345-355, titled
**'Ameliorative effects of Moringa oleifera Lam
seed extract on liver fibrosis in rats'** clearly
establishes "The activity of superoxide
dismutase as well as the content of both
malondialdehyde and protein carbonyl, which
are oxidative stress markers, were **reversed** after
treatment with Moringa. Finally, these results
suggested that Moringa seed extract can act

against CCl4-induced liver injury and fibrosis in rats by a mechanism related to its antioxidant properties, anti-inflammatory effect and its ability to **attenuate the hepatic stellate cells activation**.

In liver cirrhosis pathology, the activation of hepatic stellate cells (HSCs) is a pivotal event in fibrosis. This is a well-known fact and the above article establishes Moringa's ability to attenuate the hepatic stellate cell activation.

Phyllanthus niruri

A study by Zahra A. Amin et al titled **"Protective Role of Phyllanthus niruri Extract against Thioacetamide-Induced Liver Cirrhosis in Rat Model'** published in Evidence-Based Complementary and Alternative Medicine, Volume 2012, Article ID 241583, 9 pages
The abstract of this article states that "Histopathological analysis revealed necrosis, lymphocytes infiltration in the centrilobular region, and fibrous connective tissue proliferation in the livers of the hepatotoxic rats. But, the livers of the treated rats had comparatively minimal inflammation and normal lobular architecture. Silymarin and

Phyllanthus niruri treatments **effectively restored these measurements closer to their normal levels**. Progression of liver cirrhosis induced by TAA in rats can be intervened using the Phyllanthus niruri extract and these effects are comparable to those of silymarin"

Picrorhiza kurroa

A study by Sapna N Shetty et al titled "**A study of standardized extracts of Picrorhiza kurroa Royle ex Benth in experimental nonalcoholic fatty liver disease**" is Published in 'Journal of Ayurveda and integrated medicine', 2010 Jul-Sep; 1(3): 203–210.
The study establishes with evidence "Compared to the standard dose of the known hepatoprotective silymarin, P. kurroa reduced the lipid content (mg/g) of the liver more significantly at the dose of 400mg/kg (57.71 ± 12.45mg/kg vs. 29.44 ± 8.49 for the silymarin group vs. 400mg/kg of P. kurroa, P<0.001). In view of the increasing prevalence of metabolic syndrome and NAFLD, P. kurroa should be investigated by the reverse pharmacology path as a potential drug for the treatment of NAFLD(Non-Alcoholic Fatty Liver Disease)

Boerhavia Diffusa
A study by M.V Patel titled "**A Complex Multiherbal Regimen Based on Ayurveda**

Medicine for the Management of Hepatic Cirrhosis Complicated by Ascites: Nonrandomized, Uncontrolled, Single Group, Open-Label Observational Clinical Study" is published in 'Evidence-Based Complementary and Alternative Medicine', Volume 2015, Article ID 613182.

The study establishes the general potential of Ayurvedic therapy for overall clinical outcomes in hepatic cirrhosis complicated by ascites (HCcA). In form of a nonrandomized, uncontrolled, single group, open-label observational clinical study, 56 patients fulfilling standardized diagnostic criteria for HCcA were observed during their treatment at the P. D. Patel Ayurveda Hospital, Nadiad, India. Based on Ayurvedic tradition, a standardized treatment protocol was developed and implemented, consisting of oral administration of single and compound herbal preparations combined with purificatory measures as well as dietary and lifestyle regimens. The outcomes were assessed by measuring liver functions through specific clinical features and laboratory parameters and by evaluating the Child-Pugh prognostic grade score. After 6 weeks of treatment and a follow-up period of 18 weeks, the outcomes showed statistically significant and clinically relevant improvements. Further larger and randomized trials on the effectiveness, safety, and quality of the Ayurvedic approach in the treatment of HCcA are guaranteed to support these preliminary findings.

Tinospora cordifolia
A study by DS Nagarkatti et al, titled **'Modulation of Kupffer cell activity by Tinospora cordifolia in liver damage'** published in "Journal of Postgraduate Medicine" 1994 Apr-Jun;40(2):65-7.

Abstract of the study

Kupffer cells are major determinants of outcome of liver injury. Their activity was therefore studied in a model of chronic liver disease. The effect of Tinospora cordifolia, an indigenous agent with proven hepatoprotective activity, was evaluated on Kupffer cell function, using carbon clearance test as a parameter. Rats were divided into two major groups. In Gp I which served as normal control t1/2 of carbon was 9.48 +/- 4.14 min. GpII received horse-serum in a dose of 0.5 ml/100 gm b.w. i.p. for a period of 12 weeks and was divided into three sub-groups. In Gp IIA at the end of 12 weeks, the half-life of carbon was found to be significantly increased to 19.86 +/- 7.95 min (p < 0.01). Indicating suppressed Kupffer cell function in chronic liver damage. In Gp IIB treated with vehicle for 4 more weeks, there was a significant prolongation of half-life to 38.32 +/- 10.61 min (p < 0.01), indicating perpetuation of damage in absence of the damaging agent. Whereas in Gp IIc, treated with Tinospora cordifolia t 1/2 was decreased to 14.24 7.74 min (p < .01), as compared to vehicle control indicating a significant improvement in Kupffer cell function **and a trend towards normalization**.

In addition to all the information above, the below study sheds light to the interplay between gut microbiota and herbal medicines.

A study by j. Xu et al titled "Understanding the Molecular Mechanisms of the Interplay Between Herbal Medicines and Gut Microbiota" published in 'Medical Research Reviews', Volume37, Issue5, September 2017, Pages 1140-1185.

Abstract of the study

Herbal medicines (HMs) are much appreciated for their significant contribution to human survival and reproduction by remedial and prophylactic management of diseases. Defining the scientific basis of HMs will substantiate their value and promote their modernization. Ever-increasing evidence suggests that gut microbiota plays a crucial role in HM therapy by complicated interplay with HM components. This interplay includes such activities as: gut microbiota biotransforming HM chemicals into metabolites that harbor different bioavailability and bioactivity/toxicity from their precursors; HM chemicals improving the composition of gut microbiota, consequently ameliorating its dysfunction as well as associated pathological conditions; and gut microbiota mediating the interactions (synergistic and antagonistic) between the multiple chemicals in HMs. More advanced experimental designs are recommended for future studies, such as overall chemical characterization of gut microbiota-metabolized HMs, direct microbial analysis of HM-targeted gut microbiota, and precise gut microbiota research model development. The outcomes of such research can further elucidate the interactions between HMs and gut microbiota, thereby opening a new window for defining the scientific basis of HMs and for guiding HM-based drug discovery.

What is your contribution to this treatment?

I have no contribution to this treatment or diet plan since this has been followed since ancient times. On top of this information, reputed herbal medicine experts in India like **expertayurveda.com** and **planetayurveda.com** sell these combinations of herbs to treat liver cirrhosis and there are hundreds of patients reversed their cirrhosis with herbal medicines alone. Many of these herbalists are treating this condition without knowing much about the microbiome but in my journey, I was lucky to meet some of the seers in south India, who got more in-depth knowledge about this gut flora and they manipulate it with different herbal media. They give me the idea about diet restrictions and the special diet that was described in my book and this has been practiced and prescribed by many in the country. My earnest attempt is to shed light on the direct relation of this treatment with recent scientific advances.

What is the key rule in this treatment?

Normally, you will get a new liver every six weeks. That is how fast liver can regenerate but, what we need is beneficial microbes to provide enough nutrients for this to happen. Hence, the key rule in this treatment is feeding the beneficial microbes alone by taking the special diet and herbs as discussed in chapter 3 and maintaining your body temperature (chapter 2). Also, calming your mind with meditation would all adds to a speedy recovery. In a nutshell, diet restriction with herbal supplements and special diet is the key to this treatment.

5. FAQs and Conclusion

Can I sleep during the daytime?

No, if possible. It is hard for most liver cirrhosis patients to sleep during night time. But, sleeping during the daytime after we take food is not recommended at least for 2 hours as this may adversely affect your digestion. When you sleep, the temperature of your body comes down, and this together with food in your stomach would favor pathogens to thrive. Showers should also be in warm water to maintain the body temperature, and it is imperative to avoid showers within two hours of food for the same reason.

Do I still need to take medication by my gastroenterologist?

You need to take all prescribed medication by your concerned gastroenterologist. Once the symptoms subside, you can entirely rely on the diet plan and herbal medications, but as I mentioned in the above question, this will take 15 to 30 days to see any changes. You may still need to take medicines for ascites and portal hypertension for some more time till your albumin levels are up, or your INR is close to normal. Do not mix your regular medicines with the herbal ones. Try to keep at least an hour gap between them. The reason is beneficial microbes do not prefer chemicals as their medium.

I take medication for diabetes. Do I need to stop it?

Not at all. Sugar levels need to be entirely under control throughout this treatment. Pathogens love excess sugar in the bloodstream, and many of the diseases including liver cirrhosis get worse by uncontrolled sugar levels. Always monitor your glucose levels and take medications accordingly. However, as you progress with the treatment plan, you can see your sugar levels coming down, in that case, you need to adjust your diabetes medication dose otherwise there are chances that you may go hypoglycemic. Always be under the supervision of your medical practitioner with doses of your regular medications. Further, it is not recommended to mix these herbal medicines with your regular ones. Take at least an hour gap between the two.

Why is grass-fed butter or cold pressed coconut oil or olive oil is important in this treatment?

It is quite evident from recent researches that cold pressed coconut oil or grass-fed butter contains fat-soluble phytochemicals which are not lost by the process of heating. It is incredibly important for this treatment since what stops the pathogens to multiply is the phytochemicals; making the food a bad medium for the pathogens, but beneficial ones thrive in it. Remember: do not heat this oil or fat at any circumstances.

Why all these herbal medicines?

All those herbal medicines[iv,v,vi] retain all natural chemicals, and even they are in very minimal quantities they are potent enough to make the whole system a better medium to beneficial microbes. Moreover, this situation needs intensive treatment to get the best out of it. Among those herbs, some are rejuvenating; many are cleansing. A complete profile of each herb is not the intent of this book, but overall they are very potent mediums for beneficial microbes.

What to check for when buying these herbal medicines?

The very primary thing to check for while buying these herbs is its ingredients. Each herb should be pure and organic if possible. There shouldn't be any preservatives or additives in it. If you can get sun-dried ones that are even better since it retains the most natural nutrients. If you are lucky organic sun-dried pure herbs are the ones to get the best results.

How long do I need to take these herbal medicines and diet plan?

If you could start all the herbal medicines, you can see changes as early as 15 days to a month. If you continue with this over 90 days with all the parameters under control which are mentioned in chapter 2, you would have reversed your liver cirrhosis. If still recovering, continue with the treatment and herbal medicine for another 90 days. In between, if you find any difficulties, with no reluctance contact your gastroenterologist at the earliest.

<u>*Conclusion*</u>

The entire cure procedure was used exclusively for maintaining the body to proceed with the spiritual pursuits during ancient times. The seers used to have more potent herbs like a variety of somalata that went extinct over time. Although this seems to be an intensive procedure, once you get all prescribed herbs, things would go much easier. The results of this treatment and diet plan outweigh its intensity or other diet restrictions. It is inevitable to stick with your regular medicines until you find yourself manageable with these herbal ones. As described in the subject once you properly colonize the beneficial ones, you can change to your normal diet but completely avoid alcohol, smoking and junk food as now you know the real causes of your disease. 90 days is the minimum to get cirrhosis reversed, but if the parameters mentioned in chapter 2, is not under control, you may need 180 days or even more.

6. References

[i] A. Alexopoulou, Bacterial translocation markers in liver cirrhosis, Ann Gastroenterol. 2017; 30(5): 486–497, Published online 2017 Jul 25, DOI: **10.20524/aog.2017.0178**

[ii] R. Cabrera-Rubio. The human milk microbiome changes over lactation and is shaped by maternal weight and mode of delivery. American Journal of Clinical Nutrition, 2012; 96 (3): 544 DOI: **10.3945/ajcn.112.037382**

[iii] Lönnerdal B, Effects of maternal dietary intake on human milk composition. Journal of Nutrition.1986, Apr Apr;116(4):499-513. **10.1093/jn/116.4.499**

[iv] Gosh N, Recent advances in herbal medicine for treatment of liver diseases, Pharm Biol. 2011 Sep;49(9):970-88, doi: 10.3109/13880209.2011.558515

[v] J Xiao, Recent Advances in the Herbal Treatment of Non-Alcoholic Fatty Liver Disease, Journal of Traditional and Complementary Medicine, Volume 3, Issue 2, April–June 2013, pages 88-94.

[vi] S Chen, Potent natural products and herbal medicines for treating liver fibrosis, Chin Med. 2015; 10: 7. Published online 2015 Apr 15,doi: **10.1186/s13020-015-0036-y**

www.ingramcontent.com/pod-product-compliance
Lightning Source LLC
Chambersburg PA
CBHW051132250726
48655CB00007B/3015